THE CRY OF MY BABY

STEP BY STEP TREATMENT FOR INFERTILITY

WELCOME A BABY AFTER DECADES

A baby is the pride of the mother

Dr Ben JAPHETH

TABLE OF CONTENTS

INTRODUCTION

Chapter 1

TYPES OF INFERTILITY

Chapter 2

HOW TO CONTROL INFERTILITY

- MAINTAINING A NORMAL BODY WEIGHT

- GO FOR EXERCISE

- DON'T SMOKE

- DON'T HAVE UNPROTECTED SEX

- ANTIBIOTICS FOR TREATING INFERTILITY

Chapter 3

HOW TO BOOST FERTILITY IN WOMEN

HOW TO BOOST FERTILITY IN MEN

Chapter 4

COULD A CHANGE OF ENVIRONMENT AFFECT INFERTILITY

Encouragement

INTRODUCTION

<u>INFERTILITY IN MARRIAGE</u>

Gravidity, defined as the incapability to conceive a child after one time of vulnerable intercourse, is a global health issue affecting millions of couples. According to the World Health Organization(WHO), roughly 10 to 15 of couples encyclopedia all witness gravidity, with this number adding over the times. Gravidity can have significant cerebral, emotional, and social consequences on couples, including depression, anxiety, and social insulation.

This essay will bandy the causes, opinion, and operation of gravidity.

Gravidity can be caused by a variety of factors, including inheritable, physiological, and environmental factors. One of the most common causes of gravidity is age.

As women age, their ovarian reserve, which Is the number of eggs the ovaries can produce, decreases, leading to a drop in fertility.

In men, age also affects fertility since the quality, volume, and motility of sperm decreases with age.

Other physiological factors that can beget gravidity include hormonal imbalances, polycystic ovary pattern(PCOS), endometriosis, and tubal obstructions.

inheritable factors similar to abnormal chromosomes or inheritable mutations can also contribute to gravidity.

Environmental factors similar as exposure to poisonous substances, alcohol, and cigarette smoking can also affect fertility, and it's recommended to avoid these factors when trying to conceive.

Diagnosing gravidity generally involves a comprehensive medical evaluation of both mates, including physical examinations, medical history, and laboratory testing.

Depending on the results of these evaluations, further testing similar as ultrasounds, hysterosalpingography, or semen analysis may be conducted.

Gravidity can be managed through a variety of means depending on the underpinning cause.

For illustration, hormonal imbalances can be treated with specifics similar to clomiphene citrate,gonadotropins to stimulate ovulation in women.

In men, testosterone supplements may be specified to ameliorate sperm quality and motility.

In cases of severe manly gravidity, in vitro fertilization(IVF) or intracytoplasmic sperm injection(ICSI) may be recommended.

For women with tubal obstructions or endometriosis, surgery may be necessary to ameliorate fertility.

In vitro fertilization(IVF) is a generally used supported reproductive technology(ART) that involves reacquiring eggs from a woman's ovaries and fertilizing them with sperm in a laboratory.

The performing embryos are also transferred back to the woman's uterus with the stopgap of a successful gestation.

In some cases, life changes similar to weight loss, quitting smoking and reducing alcohol input may also ameliorate a couple's chances of conceiving. In conclusion, gravidity is a significant health issue affecting millions of couples worldwide and can have severe cerebral and emotional consequences.

Causes of gravidity range from inheritable and physiological factors to environmental and life factors.

A comprehensive medical evaluation is necessary to diagnose gravidity and determine the stylish course of treatment.

Advances in ART, similar to IVF and ICSI, have proven successful in perfecting fertility for numerous couples.

Still, forestallment is always the stylish course, and couples should aim to borrow healthy cultures and limit exposure to poisons and dangerous substances.

Types of infertility

Conceive after one time of sexual intercourse without the use of contraceptive measures. Gravidity affects roughly 8- 12 of couples worldwide, with manly factors contributing in 30- 50% of cases and womanish factors contributing in 30- 50% cases; in some cases, both manly and womanish factors may be responsible.

The remaining cases of gravidity are caused by a combination of both manly and womanish factors or unknown factors. The type of gravidity can be classified into two orders – primary and secondary.

Primary gravidity refers to couples who haven't been suitable to conceive after trying for one time, while secondary gravidity refers to couples who have had a successful gestation in history but are unfit to conceive again after trying for one time. This bracket is grounded on the capability of the couple to conceive rather than their capability to carry a gestation to term. There are several reasons for gravidity.

In ladies, ovulatory dysfunction, tubal abnormalities, endometriosis, and uterine abnormalities are the most common causes of gravidity.

Ovulatory dysfunction or anovulation occurs when a woman's ovaries fail to release an egg, making it insolvable for fertilization to do.

Tubal abnormalities are caused by damage or blockages in the fallopian tubes, which help the sperm from reaching the egg.

Endometriosis is a condition where the towel that typically lines the uterus grows outside the uterus, frequently around the ovaries and fallopian tubes, causing scarring and adhesions that can block the fallopian tubes.

Uterine abnormalities, similar to fibroids or cysts, can also affect fertility by snooping with implantation of the fertilized egg. In males, the most common cause of gravidity is abnormal sperm product or function. This can be due to inheritable abnormalities, hormonal imbalances, or environmental factors similar to exposure to poisonous chemicals.

Other factors that can affect manly fertility include varicoceles, which are enlarged modes in the scrotum that can beget dropped sperm quality, and retrograde interjection, where the semen goes into the bladder rather than being exclaimed out of the penis.

In some cases, gravidity may be caused by immunological factors.

In women, antibodies can be produced against their mate's sperm, making it delicate to conceive.

In men, antibodies can be produced against their own sperm, making it delicate for the sperm to fertilize an egg.

There are also some other less common causes of gravidity, similar as certain medical conditions like diabetes or thyroid problems, exposure to radiation or chemotherapy, and certain specifics that can intrude with fertility.
Gravidity can be diagnosed through several tests and examinations.

In women, tests similar to blood tests to measure hormone situations, ultrasound reviews to fantasize the uterus and ovaries, and hysterosalpingography, which is a color test to check the fallopian tubes, can be done.

Other tests similar as laparoscopy and hysteroscopy may also be done to probe any beginning abnormalities.
In men, semen analysis is generally the first test that's done to check for abnormalities in sperm count, motility, and morphology.
Treatment for gravidity depends on the cause of the problem.

In some cases, life changes similar to weight loss, quitting smoking, or reducing alcohol consumption can ameliorate fertility. Specifics can also be specified to help women with ovulatory dysfunction, or to ameliorate manly sperm quality.

supported reproductive ways similar as intrauterine copulation(IUI) or in vitro fertilization(IVF) may also be recommended depending on the specific situation. In conclusion, gravidity can be caused by several different factors in both men and women.

Diagnosing and treating gravidity can be a complex process that requires technical knowledge and moxie.

By working with a healthcare provider who specializes in fertility, couples can develop a personalized treatment plan that can increase their chances of successfully conceiving a child.

HOW TO CONTROL INFERTILITY

- MAINTAINING A NORMAL BODY WEIGHT
- GO FOR EXERCISE
- DON'T SMOKE
- DON'T HAVE UNPROTECTED SEX
- ANTIBIOTICS FOR TREATING INFERTILITY

MAINTAINING A NORMAL BODY WEIGHT

is pivotal for a healthy life. multitudinous studies have shown that being fat or fat can lead to several health complications similar to heart conditions, diabetes, and high blood pressure. These health complications can significantly reduce life expectancy and affect the quality of life. Hence, it's consummate to maintain a healthy body weight. The first step towards maintaining a normal body weight is understanding what it means.

A normal body weight is a balance between the number of calories we consume and the quantum of energy we expend.
When we consume more calories than we expend, the redundant calories are stored in the body as fat. Within some period , it leads to weight gain.

Thus, it's important to make sure we consume just enough calories to meet our energy requirements. One way to maintain a normal body weight is to eat a balanced diet.

A balanced diet is one that consists of all the essential nutrients that the body requires in the right proportions. Here are some classes of food carbohydrates, proteins, fats, vitamins, and minerals.
A balanced diet ensures that we get all the necessary nutrients, and at the same time, we don't consume redundant calories that can lead to weight gain.
It's also important to watch our portions and limit our sugar and sodium input. Sugar and sodium are in utmost reused foods and can lead to weight gain.

By covering our portion sizes and limiting our consumption of reused foods, we can minimize our chances of getting fat or fat. Exercise is also essential for maintaining a normal body weight.
Exercise helps burn calories and increase our body's energy expenditure. Physical exertion also helps make muscles, which in turn, helps increase our metabolic rate.

This means that the further muscle we have, the further calories we burn indeed when at rest. Thus, it's essential to incorporate regular exercise into our diurnal routine.

Cardiovascular exercises similar to running, cycling and swimming are effective in burning calories when done regularly.

Resistance training similar to toning and calisthenics helps make muscles and raise metabolic rate, which aids in burning calories indeed when we aren't exercising.

Several studies have shown that sleep also plays a part in maintaining a normal body weight. Lack of sleep has been set up to be associated with weight gain and rotundity. When we don't get enough sleep, our body produces more of the hormone ghrelin, which stimulates appetite, and lower levels of the hormone leptin, which suppresses appetite. It can lead to weight gain. Also, lack of sleep can intrude with the hormones that regulate our metabolism.

Good quality sleep helps regulate these hormones, lower appetite, and ameliorate metabolism, making it easier to maintain a healthy body weight. In conclusion, maintaining a normal body weight is essential for a healthy life.

A healthy weight helps reduce the threat of several health complications similar to heart complaints, diabetes, and high blood pressure.

Eating a balanced diet, regular exercise, and getting enough sleep are essential for maintaining a normal body weight.

By covering our portion sizes, limiting our consumption of sticky and reused foods, and incorporating regular physical exertion into our routine, we can maintain a healthy body weight. Eventually, it's essential to cultivate healthy habits to live a fulfilling life.

GO FOR EXERCISE

Introduction

Preface Exercise plays a critical part in promoting health and well- being. While most people are apprehensive of the physical and internal benefits of exercise, not many understand the impact of exercise on fertility, particularly in women. Research studies have established a clear association between exercise and fertility.

Moderate to high- intensity physical exertion can boost generality chances by perfecting ovarian function, adding blood inflow to the reproductive organs, and reducing stress situations. In this essay, we will look at the types of exercises that can enhance generality in women.
Cardiovascular Exercise One of the most effective types of exercise for promoting fertility in women is cardiovascular exercise.

Cardiovascular conditioning includes running, cycling, swimming, and brisk walking. These exercises increase blood inflow to the reproductive organs, perfecting the chances of generality.

Cardiovascular exercises also boost energy situations and reduce stress situations, both of which are essential factors for promoting fertility.

Research has shown that women who engage in at least 30 twinkles of moderate- intensity cardiovascular exercise at least three times a week increase their fertility chances. Strength Training Strength training is another type of exercise that can ameliorate fertility in women.

Strength training exercises develop spare muscle mass, which boosts metabolism and helps to maintain a healthy weight. Maintaining a healthy weight is critical for fertility since being either fat or light can impact the situations of certain hormones, similar as estrogen and testosterone, that affect a woman's capability to conceive.

Resistance exercises, similar to weight lifting, squats, and lunges, can help to ameliorate balance and posture, reducing the liability of cascade or injuries that could negatively impact fertility.

Yoga Yoga is a fantastic exercise that can promote fertility and overall health in women. Yoga involves stretching, deep breathing, and relaxation ways that can help to reduce stress situations and ameliorate blood inflow to the pelvic region.

The relaxation ways and deep breathing exercises in yoga can also help to regulate hormone situations, reducing anxiety, and promoting ovulation.

rehearsing yoga postures that involve the hips, similar to the chump, butterfly, and happy baby, can help to increase blood inflow to the reproductive organs, promoting a healthy gestation.

Studies have reported that women who exercise yoga regularly witness reduced menstrual pain, regulated menstrual cycles, and increased fertility. Pilates Pilates is a type of low- impact exercise that can help to ameliorate rotation, posture, and pelvic stability.
By engaging the core muscles, Pilates exercises can help to ameliorate rotation to the reproductive organs, promoting healthy reproductive function.
Pilates exercises also help to relieve stress and increase inflexibility, which can be essential for women who are trying to conceive.

Research studies have set up that Pilates can ameliorate fertility by reducing stress situations and perfecting body composition. In conclusion, engaging in regular exercise is a pivotal factor in promoting fertility in women.

Cardiovascular exercises, similar as running, cycling, swimming, and brisk walking, help to increase blood inflow to the reproductive organs, perfecting the chances of generality.

Strength training exercises, similar to weight lifting, squats, and lunges, can ameliorate posture and balance, reducing the liability of cascade or injuries that could negatively affect fertility.

Yoga and Pilates are also effective exercises that can promote fertility by reducing stress situations, perfecting posture, and rotation and regulating hormone situations to promote ovulation. Women who are trying to conceive should consider engaging in some form of exercise to promote reproductive health.

Citations - Pivarnik,J.M., Chambliss,H.O., Clapp,J.F., Dugan,S.A., Hatch,M.C., Lovelady,C.A., & Williams,M.A.(2006).
I
mpact of physical exertion during gestation and postpartum on habitual complaint threat.
Medicine and wisdom in sports and exercise, 38(5),989-1006. - Dechanet,C., Anahory, I., Mathieu Daude,J.C., Quantin,X., Reyftmann,L., Hamamah,S., & Hedon,B.(2011). goods of cigarette smoking on reduplication.

mortal reduplication update, 17(1), 76- 95. Gravidity is a medical condition that affects numerous individualities and couples around the world. It's defined as the incapability to conceive a child after a time of vulnerable coitus.

In recent times, exercise has surfaced as a potentially salutary system to control and manage gravidity.

In this essay, we will discuss how exercise can help control gravidity and the different types of exercises that can be salutary for individuals and couples floundering with gravidity.

Exercise and gravidity have been linked in several studies. Regular exercise can ameliorate sleep quality, reduce stress, and enhance the overall health of individualities.

Exercising can also help individualities control their weight, maintain healthy blood sugar situations, and reduce the threat of colorful conditions, including PCOS(Polycystic Ovary Pattern), a leading cause of womanish gravidity.

A study published in the Journal of Clinical Endocrinology and Metabolism set up that women with PCOS who exercised regularly had bettered insulin perceptivity and hormonal balance, appreciatively impacting their chances of conceiving

DON'T SMOKE

Smoking is a significant health hazard that affects both smokers andnon-smokers. The consequences of smoking extend beyond an individual, which includes the impact on fetal and child development.

Smoking during gestation not only poses a threat to the woman's health but also to the baby's health. According to the Centers for Disease Control and Prevention(CDC), smoking during gestation can beget low birth weight, unseasonable birth and birth.

This essay will explore the benefits of smoking on child-bearing and the health of the child. Smoking during gestation can beget significant detriment to the fetus, including low birth weight. Low birth weight is defined as importing lower than 5.5 pounds at birth.

Low birth weight can have long- term consequences and is associated with health problems like high blood pressure, cardiovascular complaint, and type 2 diabetes. Studies have shown that babies whose mothers
bombs during gestation are at an advanced threat of low birth weight. Also, smoking while pregnant can also lead to preterm birth, which is defined as giving birth before 37 weeks.

Preterm birth can beget the baby to face health complications or indeed death. Smoking while pregnant also has after- goods on the baby's health after birth. Alternate- hand bank can have ruinous goods on the child's health.

According to the American Academy of Pediatrics, alternate- hand banks can beget unforeseen child death patterns(SIDS), bronchitis, asthma, and observance infections.
Indeed if parents choose not to bomb around their child, third- hand bank(residual nicotine and other chemicals left on a face from smoking) can still beget health problems for the baby.

 This threat of health issues isn't only a concern for the baby's early times but also for their long- term health. Studies have shown that children born to meters
who smoked during gestation are at an advanced threat of developing respiratory complications, including asthma. Also, these children may also have cognitive and behavioral problems.

This may increase the threat of attention deficiency hyperactivity complaint(ADHD) and other behavioral diseases. It's essential to note that smoking during gestation doesn't only pose long- term health complications for the baby but also for the mama .

According to the American Lung Association, women who bomb during gestation are at advanced threat of developing gestation complications similar as ectopic gestation, confinement, and unseasonable labor.

Women who bomb also have an advanced chance of passing fertility problems and gestation complications in unborn gravidity.
Quitting smoking during gestation can significantly reduce the threat of health problems, indeed if conclusion occurs latterly in the gestation.
Smoking during gestation can have long- term health effects on children.
Exploration shows that children whose parents bomb are at advanced threat of developing lung cancer and heart complaints in majority.
Children who grow up in homes with smokers are also more likely to become smokers. This is because they're more likely to model the geste
they see around them.

 Also, smoking during gestation can have a considerable profitable impact on families. Low birth weight and unseasonable birth can beget a baby to spend extended ages in the sanitarium, leading to significant medical bills.

Also, children with asthma or other health issues associated with smoking may bear further medical attention, which can also be economically burdensome for families.

In conclusion, smoking during gestation can have long-lasting mischievous goods on the health of the mama and child. Smoking while pregnant can beget low birth weight, preterm birth, and health complications in the child.

These health complications can extend into the child's adolescent and adult times, leading to an increased threat of respiratory problems and cognitive/ behavioral issues. Pregnant maters
who quit smoking can significantly reduce the threat of their own and their child's health issues.

The medical and profitable consequences of smoking during gestation make it a vital issue to address in public health converse.

UNPROTECTED SEX

Vulnerable coitus, also known as coitus without the use of contraception, can lead to a range of negative health issues. One of the most serious consequences can be gravidity. Gravidity is defined as the incapability to conceive a child after one time of vulnerable intercourse.

It can be caused by a range of factors, including age, medical conditions, and life factors.
Vulnerable coitus can increase the threat of gravidity in both men and women, and it's important for individuals to understand the pitfalls associated with this geste .

One of the main ways vulnerable coitus can lead to gravidity is by adding the threat of sexually transmitted infections(STIs).

STIs can beget damage to the reproductive system, leading to scarring, inflammation, and other problems that can intrude with fertility.

For illustration, chlamydia and gonorrhea are two common STIs that can beget pelvic seditious complaints(PID).
PID is a serious infection of the reproductive organs that can lead to scarring, blockages, and other complications that can make it delicate or insolvable to conceive a child.

Women who have had undressed chlamydia or gonorrhea are also at advanced threat of passing gestation complications, similar as ectopic gestation or confinement.

In addition to STIs, vulnerable coitus can also increase the threat of unintended gestation, which can have a range of negative health consequences.

For illustration, unintended gestation can lead to high blood pressure, gravid diabetes, and other complications that can affect the health of both the mama and the baby.
 Also, unintended gestation can lead to a detention in seeking antenatal
care, which can further increase the threat of complications and negatively impact fetal development.

There are also a range of life factors that can impact fertility, and vulnerable coitus can increase the threat of exposure to these factors.

For illustration, smoking and medicine use can have a negative impact on fertility, and individualities who engage in these actions may be more likely to have vulnerable coitus.

Also, certain environmental factors, such as exposure to fungicides and other chemicals, can also impact fertility, and individualities who have vulnerable coitus may be at an advanced threat of exposure.

It's important for individuals to take away their fertility by using contraception and rehearsing safe coitus.

Condoms are one of the most effective forms of contraception for guarding against STIs and unintended gestation.
They work by creating a hedge that prevents sperm, STIs, and other fluids from entering the body.
Other forms of contraception, similar as the lozenge, patch, or intrauterine device(IUD), can also be effective at precluding unintended gestation, but they don't give protection against STIs.
In addition to using contraception, individualities can also reduce their threat of gravidity by making healthy life choices.
This includes avoiding smoking and medicine use, maintaining a healthy weight, and limiting exposure to environmental poisons.

It's also important for individualities to seek medical care if they suspect they may have an STI or another medical condition that could impact their fertility.

In conclusion, vulnerable coitus can have serious consequences for fertility.
individuals who engage in vulnerable coitus are at increased threat of STIs, unintended gestation, and exposure to life and environmental factors that can impact fertility.

It's important for individuals to take away their fertility by using contraception, rehearsing safe coitus, and making healthy life choices.
By taking these ways, individualities can reduce their threat of gravidity and ameliorate their overall reproductive health.

ANTIBIOTICS IN TREATING INFERTILITY

The World Health Organization(WHO) reports that gravity affects roughly 48.5 million couples encyclopedia ally.

Gravidity is characterized as the incapability of a couple to conceive after 12 months of vulnerable intercourse.

The causes of gravidity can be varied and complex, including factors similar to the age of the couple, inheritable diseases, life, and environmental factors.

Antibiotics aren't generally employed in the treatment of gravidity, but there's adding interest in studying the implicit efficacy of antibiotics in this environment.

Antibiotics are a type of drug that fights bacterial infections by either killing bacteria or decelerating their growth.

These medicines are generally specified in situations where bacteria have infected an individual and caused an illness.

Still, some exploration has suggested that antibiotics could be used to treat gravidity when it's caused by an underpinning bacterial infection.

The bacterial group Mycoplasma genitalium has been linked as an implicit cause of gravidity.M. genitalium is a sexually transmitted bacterium and is estimated to beget up to 20% of urethritis cases in men and women.

Still, the bacterium frequently goes undiagnosed due to a lack of accurate individual tools. also, there's substantiation thatM. genitalium can also beget pelvic seditious complaint(PID), a condition linked to gravidity in women. A study published in the New England Journal of Medicine on the treatment ofM. genitalium showed promising results.

Of the 186 men and women sharing in the study, half entered azithromycin, an antibiotic generally used to treat bacterial infections, while the other half entered a placebo.

In the group that entered azithromycin, 71 had noM. genitalium detected in their genital samples after three weeks, compared to only 31 in the placebo group.

This study suggests that antibiotics could potentially be an effective treatment for gravidity caused byM. genitalium.

Another implicit cause of gravidity is Chlamydia trachomatis, a bacteria that's a common cause of sexually transmitted infections(STIs). In women, Chlamydia trachomatis can lead to PID, which can beget gravidity.

Although Chlamydia trachomatis can be treated with antibiotics similar to azithromycin, exploration suggests that indeed after successful treatment, women may remain at an increased threat of PID and gravidity.

In a study published in the Journal of Infectious conditions, experimenters set up that women who were successfully treated for Chlamydia trachomatis were over four times more likely to develop PID compared to women who had Chlamydia trachomatis.

This suggests that the treatment of infections with Chlamydia trachomatis may not guarantee a reduced threat of gravidity caused by PID.

While antibiotics show implicit as a treatment for gravidity caused by bacterial infections, there are limitations and implicit side goods that must be considered.

Overuse of antibiotics can lead to antibiotic resistance, which is a growing issue worldwide. Likewise, indeed if antibiotics successfully treat the infection, there's no guarantee that fertility will be restored.

Also, the long- term goods of antibiotics on the microbiome aren't completely understood and may potentially be detrimental.

In conclusion, while antibiotics aren't the primary treatment for gravidity, they've shown implicit in treating infections that beget gravidity.

It's essential to consider the underpinning cause of gravidity before deciding on the stylish course of action, as antibiotics may not be applicable for all cases.

Also, it's important to consider the implicit pitfalls associated with overuse of antibiotics in the environment of treating gravidity.

further exploration is necessary to completely understand the implicit part of antibiotics in treating gravidity.

Citations - Jensen,J.S., Bradshaw,C.S., Tabrizi,S.N., Fairley,C.K., Hamasuna,R., Saito,S.,. & Taylor-Robinson,D.(2019). Azithromycin Treatment for Mycoplasma genitalium-Positive Urethritis and Cervicitis: A Randomized Controlled Trial.

New England Journal of Medicine, 380(10), 909- 917. - Ness,R.B., Soper,D.E., Holley,R.L., .Peipert,J., Randall,H., Sweet,R.L.,. & Hendrix,S.L.(2004). Effectiveness of outpatient and inpatient treatment strategies for women with pelvic seditious complaint Results from the Pelvic seditious complaint Evaluation and Clinical Health(PEACH) Randomized Trial. Journal of Infectious conditions, 189(4), 647- 657.

HOW TO BOOST FERTILITY IN WOMEN

Fertility is a central concern for numerous women. Whether they're trying to conceive or simply wanting to maintain their reproductive health, the content of fertility is frequently at the top of their minds. Fortunately, there are colorful ways to boost fertility in women that are both effective and safe.
One of the most critical factors in womanish fertility is maintaining a healthy weight.

Being fat or fat can lead to hormonal imbalances, which can significantly vitiate a woman's capability to conceive. Again, being light can also have negative goods on fertility, as it can disrupt hormonal balance and intrude with ovulation.

Thus, women who are trying to boost their fertility should aim to maintain a healthy weight through a balanced and nutritional diet and regular exercise.

Another essential factor in promoting fertility is getting enough sleep. Sleep privation can intrude with the delicate balance of hormones that's necessary for generality, so it's pivotal to get enough sleep each night. Women who struggle with wakefulness or other sleep disturbances should consider strategies similar to establishing a regular sleep routine, rehearsing relaxation ways, and avoiding caffeine and defenses before bedtime.

Stress can also be a significant handicap to fertility, as it can disrupt the hormonal balance necessary for generality.

Women who are trying to boost their fertility should prioritize stress operation ways similar to contemplation, deep breathing, and yoga. also, engaging in conditioning that bring joy and relaxation, similar as reading, spending time outside, or connecting with loved bones

, can help to reduce stress situations and ameliorate reproductive health.

In addition to life factors, there are also several supplements that can help to promote fertility in women.

One of the most important supplements for womanish fertility is folic acid, which can help to help birth blights and may also ameliorate fertility by enhancing ovulation.

Other supplements that may be salutary for fertility include vitamin D, which can help to regulate hormones and ameliorate egg quality, and omega- 3 adipose acids, which may ameliorate the health of the ovaries and promote fertility.

For women who are floundering with fertility, there are also colorful medical and technological interventions that can help.

For illustration, fertility medicines may be specified to stimulate ovulation, while supported reproductive technologies similar as in vitro fertilization(IVF) can help to overcome other obstacles to generality.

Still, it's essential to flash back that these interventions should be used under the guidance of a trained medical professional and that they may not be applicable or effective for every woman.
In addition to these specific strategies, there are also several broader life changes that women can make to boost their fertility.

For illustration, quitting smoking and reducing alcohol consumption can ameliorate reproductive health by reducing the threat of hormonal imbalances and other fertility- related conditions.
Likewise, avoiding exposure to poisons in the terrain, similar to fungicides and chemicals set up in certain plastics, can help to cover fertility and reproductive health.
In conclusion, there are numerous ways to boost fertility in women that are both effective and safe.
By prioritizing a healthy life, stress operation, and proper supplementation, women can ameliorate their chances of generality and maintain their reproductive health for times to come.
Of course, every woman's situation is unique, so it's essential to work with a good healthcare professional to develop a substantiated plan for promoting fertility and icing overall heartiness.

HOW TO BOOST FERTILITY IN MEN

Gravidity affects millions of couples worldwide, and mainly factor gravidity makes up a significant chance of cases. Low sperm count or poor sperm quality is frequently the cause of manly gravidity.

Fortunately, there are colorful styles to boost sperm count and ameliorate sperm quality in men.

Originally, maintaining a healthy life is an essential starting point to boosting sperm.

A study conducted by Centers for Disease Control and Prevention(CDC) set up that smoking, rotundity, and inordinate alcohol consumption are some of the significant threat factors for low sperm count and poor sperm quality.

Sperm is largely sensitive to environmental factors, and exposing it to poisons like cigarette banks, alcohol, and some chemicals can negatively impact its quality and volume.

Thus, quitting smoking, reducing alcohol consumption, and maintaining a healthy body weight are pivotal factors in perfecting sperm health.

Secondly, a nutritional diet is essential for perfecting sperm health.

According to a study conducted by the American Society of Andrology, men who consume a diet rich in antioxidants like Vitamin C, Vitamin E, and beta-carotene had better sperm quality than those who did not.

Similar vitamins and nutrients, which are abundant in fruits and vegetables, cover sperm from oxidative stress, promoting healthy sperm count and perfecting sperm's motility.
Including foods similar as spinach, carrots, citrus fruits, nuts, and seafood in your diet can increase the input of essential vitamins and nutrients, perfecting overall sperm health.
Thirdly, exercise is critical for perfecting sperm health. While a sedentary life can lead to health problems that contribute to poor sperm quality, regular exercise has been shown to increase testosterone situations, which improves sperm product.

A study published in the American Journal of Lifestyle Medicine points out that men who exercise regularly have significantly advanced sperm counts, advanced sperm motility rates, and better sperm attention than those who did not. still, inordinate exercise or violent work- eschewal administrations that reach fatigue situations can have the contrary effect.

Thus, moderate exercise that includes resistance training, cardio, and stretching can have a positive impact on sperm health. Fourthly, it's essential to keep the testicles cool.

Elevated testicular temperature leads to a reduction in sperm count and quality.

This is why the testicles are located on the outside of the body, which keeps them cooler than the body's core temperature.

Several studies have set up that inordinate heat exposure to the testes for dragged ages can cause the quality and volume of sperm to decline.

Thus, it's essential to avoid conditioning that leads to testicular heating, similar to using hot barrels, sitting for extended ages, or wearing tight undergarments. Incipiently, keep stress situations in check.

High situations of stress detect the product of cortisol, a hormone that can reduce sperm count and quality.

A study published in the Fertility and Sterility Journal set up that men under high- stress situations were 47 more likely to witness low sperm count than men who weren't stressed. ways similar as awareness, yoga, regular exercise, and acupuncture can help reduce stress and boost sperm health.

In conclusion, several factors affect sperm health, but with harmonious trouble, it's possible to ameliorate both sperm quality and volume.

By maintaining a healthy weight, consuming a nutrient-rich diet, regular exercise, keeping testicle temperature cool, and reducing stress situations, men can increase their chances of perfecting sperm health.

By enforcing these simple yet effective measures, men can take charge of their reproductive health and increase their chances of generality.

Could a change of environment cause infertility?

The terrain encompasses colorful factors similar as water, air, and soil quality, radiation, temperature, and other 0 environmental adulterants that affect mortal health.

Changes to the terrain can have colorful issues on mortal health, including the capability to bear children and gravidity. Gravidity is a common condition that millions of couples witness worldwide, with colorful factors intertwined in its occasion.

The issue of whether a change in the terrain can beget gravidity is a critical concern, especially given the continued declination of our terrain. Studies indicate that there has been an increase in gravidity cases encyclopedia ally.

Gravidity can be caused by several factors, such as physiological and anatomical abnormalities, inheritable predilection, environmental adulterants, exposure to radiation, infections, and life factors, among others.

While the colorful factors causing gravidity have been well- established, the part played by changes in the terrain is a content of continued exploration and debate.

Environmental adulterants play a pivotal part in the occasion of gravidity, and the ever- adding situations of environmental toxin have a significant impact on mortal health.

Exposure to environmental adulterants similar to lead, cadmium, and mercury is common in utmost advanced countries.

For example, lead, a heavy essence present in air, water, and soil, can reduce the number of sperm produced by the manly reproductive system, leading to gravidity.

Also, exposure to fungicides and other agrarian chemicals can affect the reproductive health of individuals spending dragged ages in agrarian settings, similar to growers. Temperature is another environmental factor that could play a part in gravidity.

Climate change is allowed
to affect mortal health in colorful ways, including the reproductive system's functionality. Studies have associated increased atmospheric temperatures with the reduction in mortal reproductive capability.

An increase in temperature frequently leads to heat stress, which has been shown to reduce the number of sperm and vitiate the quality of semen.

Heat stress has also been linked with an increase in the frequency of erectile dysfunction, which could eventually lead to gravidity.
Likewise, radiation from sources like x-ray machines, microwave oven ranges, or radioactive substances used in colorful artificial and medical procedures, among others, has been linked as a cause of gravidity. For example, frequent radiation exposure can beget endless damage to the reproductive system, leading to gravidity.

Also, radiation exposure during gestation can beget fetal abnormalities that could affect natural disabilities or gravidity later in the child's life.
While there's no distrust that the terrain can beget gravidity, the extent of the influence is still unclear.
Studies in this area have been hindered by the difficulty in segregating the goods of the terrain from other factors that could contribute to gravidity.

For illustration, to determine whether environmental poisons are responsible for gravidity, one would need to control for factors similar as age, life choices, and inheritable predilection.
In conclusion, the terrain can beget gravidity through colorful factors similar as exposure to environmental adulterants, radiation, and changes in temperature.

Still, definitive studies are demanded to understand the extent of the terrain's part in gravidity.
further exploration should look at inheritable predilection, age, and other factors that may contribute to gravidity.
Also, sweats should be made to reduce environmental poisons to alleviate their dangerous goods and help gravidity.

It's critical to fete the part played by the terrain in the development of gravidity to help the continued declination of the terrain and the attendant impact on mortal health.

GET PREGNANT THROUGH IUI SUPPORT

Introduction

IUI(Intrauterine Insemination) is a form of supported reproductive technology that has come increasingly popular in recent times as a result of gravidity.

While the procedure is non-invasive compared with other fertility treatments, it still involves a thorough understanding of the process for couples looking to use IUI.

This essay will detail what IUI gestation is, how it works, the success rates, pitfalls, and benefits of the procedure, and why it may be the answer for some couples floundering to conceive.

What's IUI? Intrauterine copulation, or IUI, is a fertility treatment procedure where sperm is placed directly into a woman's uterus to ameliorate the chances of fertilization and gestation. The sperm must be collected and reused before being placed inside the uterus.

The woman will generally take hormone injections before the procedure to help stimulate ovulation and increase the chances of fertilization.

How Does IUI Work? The sperm is prepared in a laboratory, which may include washing it to exclude any undesirable accouterments and concentrate the healthy bones
. After processing, the sperm are also placed inside a catheter, which is also fitted directly into the uterus.

This placement timing generally coincides with the woman's rich window, as determined by ovulation timing or an ovulation test tackle.

This process, in combination with hormone injections, increases the liability of the sperm successfully fertilizing an egg.

The copulation itself generally takes only a few twinkles, and while it may be uncomfortable, it isn't generally painful for the woman.

Success Rates Success rates for IUI gestation are frequently delicate to generalize, but multiple factors contribute to a successful gestation. The woman's age, uterus health, and sperm quality, among other factors, can contribute to the success of IUI.

On average, one in four couples will have a pregnancy following IUI treatment and roughly 80% of those will die within three treatment cycles.

According to one study, IUI success rates are loftiest for women under 35. Pitfalls and Benefits of IUI IUI is a fairly low- threat and non-invasive procedure, with some implicit benefits, but there are still some pitfalls which must be taken into account.

One threat is the possibility of multiple gravities(having halves, triumvirates, or further), which can affect the ovulation stimulation and the placement timing of the sperm in the uterus.

Also, statistically speaking, IUI results in lower success rates for women with lower egg reserve situations or blocked fallopian tubes.

On the other hand, IUI can be much less precious than other fertility treatments numerous couples can go multiple cycles, making it an affordable and accessible option.

Also, IUI is more controlled than natural generality because the sperm is directly placed into the uterus, increasing the chances of fertilization.

Why Choose IUI? IUI may be a desirable treatment option for couples who have difficulty conceiving naturally due to issues similar as low sperm count in the mate, problems with ovulation, unexplained gravidity, or issues with cervical mucus. Also, IUI can be an excellent treatment option for lesbian couples and single women seeking fertility backing because it mimics the natural process of generality.

IUI can also be a charming treatment option for couples who prefer less invasive treatments and desire to avoid the more complex IVF procedures. Conclusion IUI gestation may be the answer for couples floundering to conceive.
   IUI is a less invasive,non-intrusive fertility treatment option that can be accessible and affordable.

 While it may not be the right answer for all couples, for those who are floundering to conceive because of specific scripts, it may be an option with high success rates.

On average, IUI gestation results in roughly 25% success rates, although factors like the mama 's age and sperm quality can play a significant factor in the success of this procedure.

The benefits of IUI include affordability and availability, making it an option for couples who can not go to more invasive or precious fertility treatments.

IUI has some pitfalls, including the possibility of multiple gravities, and it may not be the right choice for those with blocked fallopian tubes or low egg reserve.

Still, for couples dealing with other fertility issues, IUI gestation has demonstrated a lot of success in treating gravidity over the last many times.

DIFFERENCE BETWEEN IUI AND IVF SUPPORT FOR INFERTILITY

In recent times, supported reproductive technologies(ART) have increased in fashionability and have proven to be successful in helping couples achieve their parenting dreams.
Two ART procedures generally used are Intrauterine Copulation(IUI) and In Vitro Fertilization(IVF).

Although both procedures have the same overall thing, the styles used and the position of involvement differ extensively.
 In this essay, we will explore the differences between IUI and IVF.
To begin with, IUI is an introductory ART procedure that involves the insertion of concentrated sperm directly into the uterus.

To ensure the sperm are healthy, the sperm is washed and centrifuged to exclude dead or abnormal sperm.
Once this procedure is completed, the concentrated sperm is fitted into the uterus to ameliorate the chances of fertilization.

IUI is a lower position ART procedure and is generally the first option for couples passing gravidity.

Also, IUI is less invasive and less precious than IVF.
Another thing about IVF is that it have high level invasive and complicated process that involves the fertilization of an egg outside of the body in a laboratory.
During the IVF process, the womanish mate is given fertility medicines to promote the product of multiple eggs.
Once the eggs are gathered, they're also fertilized with sperm in a laboratory dish.
After successful fertilization, the performing embryos are transferred to the uterus.

IVF is a largely substantiated supported reproductive technology procedure, which has an advanced success rate than IUI, making it a more precious option.
Another significant difference between IUI and IVF is the degree of involvement needed from the couple.
In IUI, the couple will need to be available on the day of the procedure.

On the other hand, for the IVF process, the couple should be prepared to put away a significant quantum of time to ensure a positive outgrowth.

This can include diurnal injections for the womanish mate, nonstop movables , and egg reclamation.

The womanish case must be covered precisely to insure the stylish and most suitable stage for harvesting the eggs.

Likewise, IVF is a complex procedure that can offer further options for couples having difficulty conceiving. IVF is the recommended option for couples who have had a history of failed IUI procedures.

IVF gives the couple options similar as inheritable testing and embryo freezing, both of which aren't available in IUI procedures.

During the IVF procedure, inheritable testing could include webbing for inheritable blights in embryos.

Embryo freezing, on the other hand, can give the option of indurating healthy embryos for use in unborn gravidity. It's essential to understand that both IUI and IVF processes have their advantages and disadvantages.

numerous cases consider their medical condition, budget, and overall time commitment to make an informed decision. Although IUI may be less invasive and less precious, it has lower success rates than IVF.

While IVF can produce further significant results, it requires further involvement, is more invasive, and is premium.

In conclusion, both IUI and IVF ART procedures are feasible options for couples who may witness fertility issues.

One determining factor couples may consider is the cost of the procedures involved.

IUI is a more affordable option, while IVF is more precious due to the cost of the laboratory procedure, multiple movables , and specifics.
Depending on the couple's reproductive health, age, and fertility history, the choice between IUI and IVF must be made in discussion with a reproductive endocrinologist.
 Understanding the differences between IUI and IVF can help couples make an informed decision and choose the ART procedure that's stylish for them. References

----

COST FOR IUI SUPPORT

Intrauterine copulation(IUI) is an supported reproductive technology(ART) that involves placing washed, concentrated sperm directly into a woman's uterus to increase the chances of fertilization.
Couples floundering with gravidity frequently consider IUI as one of the first way in their fertility treatment trip.

still, the cost of IUI can vary depending on colorful factors, similar as the position, the clinic, the medical professionals involved, and any fresh treatments demanded.
The average cost of one IUI cycle in the United States, without insurance, can range from$ 500 to$ 4,000.
This price can be deceiving, as veritably many couples achieve a gestation with just one IUI cycle. On average, couples suffer three to four IUI cycles before conceiving.
thus, cases may end up spending up to$ 12,000 to$ 16,000 on IUI.
This doesn't include the cost of specifics, which can reach up to$ 2,500 for injectable hormones.
The reason for the variation in cost is due to the differences in medical practices from clinic to clinic.
In general, conventions in metropolitan areas tend to be more precious than those located in pastoral areas. also, conventions with advanced success rates may charge further for their services.

The cost of fresh treatments, similar as ultrasound monitoring and sperm washing, can also impact the total cost of IUI. One of the primary factors impacting the cost of IUI is insurance content.

Some insurance plans may cover some or all of the costs of IUI, while others may not cover anything at all.

For those without insurance, some conventions offer abatements for military labor force or couples who pay in full outspoken.

Cases may also consider financing options, similar as medical credit cards or particular loans, to cover the costs of IUI.

Another influential factor in the cost of IUI is the quantum of drug needed to stimulate ovulation.

The drug used in IUI can range from oral specifics, similar as Clomid, to injectable hormones, similar as follicle- stimulating hormone(FSH) and mortal chorionic gonadotropin(hCG).

Injectable specifics tend to be more precious than oral specifics, ranging from$ 1,500 to$ 2,500 per cycle. also, the cost of IUI can also vary depending on the fresh procedures needed.

For illustration, if a case requires sperm reclamation or patron sperm, this will increase the cost. fresh procedures may include ultrasound monitoring, imaging tests, and bloodwork.

These tests are necessary to insure that the case is responding to the drug and that ovulation is imminent.

In conclusion, the cost of IUI can be a significant fiscal burden for couples floundering with gravidity.

still, understanding the variation in cost and what goes into an IUI cycle can help cases make informed opinions about their fertility care. Factors similar as position, clinic, drug, and fresh procedures can all impact the total cost of IUI.

Cases may want to consider insurance content or backing options to help manage the cost.

Acting as an educated case can help insure that couples get the most out of their fertility treatments while minimizing the fiscal burden.

QUANTITY OF SPERM NEEDED FOR IUI SUPPORT

The quantum of sperm needed for an IUI procedure has been a content of debate among reproductive health professionals, as there's no agreement on the optimal volume of sperm demanded.
According to the World Health Organization, a standard semen sample should contain a minimum of 15 million spermatozoa per milliliter. still, studies have shown that success rates for IUI aren't inescapably advanced with further sperm.
One study published in the Journal of Human Reproductive lores set up no significant differences in gestation rates for samples with consistence of between 5- 10 million and 20- 30 million spermatozoa per milliliter.

Another study published in the Journal of Obstetrics and Gynaecology Canada indicated that IUI success rates weren't statistically different between men with moderate oligospermia(5- 10 million sperm) and men with milder oligospermia(10- 20 million sperm).

These studies suggest that the quality and motility of the sperm, rather than the volume, may be more important factors to consider in IUI issues.

On the other hand, a study published in the journal Fertility and Sterility reported a positive correlation between the total motile sperm count(TMSC) and gestation rates in IUI.

The TMSC, which measures the total number of precipitously motile spermatozoa in a semen sample, has been proposed as a further comprehensive marker of the sperm's fertility eventuality than the attention of sperm alone.
The study set up that a TMSC of at least 2 million spermatozoa was associated with advanced gestation rates, and success rates declined significantly when the TMSC fell below this threshold.
The authors suggest that the TMSC may be a meaningful predictor of reproductive outgrowth in men with manly factor gravidity witnessing IUI.
It's worth noting that personalized care is pivotal in reproductive drug.
The optimal volume of sperm demanded for IUI depends on colorful factors similar as age, medical history, and fertility status.
A comprehensive examination and analysis of medical and reproductive records will help conform the treatment strategy for each case.
In conclusion, the optimal volume of sperm needed for a successful IUI procedure is still a subject of debate.
While some studies suggest that the quality and motility of the sperm are more critical factors to consider than the volume, others propose the total motile sperm count(

TMSC) as a meaningful predictor of reproductive outgrowth.

nevertheless, personalized case care is consummate in determining the applicable volume of sperm demanded for an IUI procedure.

WHAT CAUSES LOW SPERM COUNT

Low sperm count, also known as oligospermia, is a condition where the semen exclaimed by a man contains smaller sperm than the normal range. The World Health Organization(WHO) defines a" normal" sperm count as having at least 15 million sperm per milliliter of semen.

Sperm is essential for fertilizing a woman's egg for generality to do.

Anything below this threshold is considered low and can lead to gravidity issues in men.

While the causes of low sperm count can be varied, we will examine some generally reported reasons in this essay. One significant cause of low sperm count is hormonal imbalances.

Hormones play an essential part in sperm product, and any dislocations can impact the process. When hormone situations aren't rightly balanced or are deficient, sperm product can be lowered.

The pituitary gland secretes Follicle- stimulating hormone(FSH) and Luteinizing hormones(LH), necessary for sperm product.

When the pituitary gland is unfit to release enough of these hormones, it can lead to low sperm counts.

These hormonal imbalances can be caused by several factors, similar as rotundity, excrescences, infections, habitual illness, and genetics.
A study set up that low sperm counts identified with poor manly health hormone biographies

ENCOURAGEMENT

Gravidity can be an emotionally draining and segregating experience for couples who are floundering to conceive. Despite the advancements in medical technology, gravidity still affects numerous couples across the globe.

According to the World Health Organization(WHO), one in six couples worldwide witness some form of gravidity.

Gravidity can be a delicate and complex trip filled with ups and campo, but there's stopgap, and there are ways to stay motivated and supported throughout the trip. stimulant is essential to help gravidity couples stay positive and hopeful throughout their trip.

Words of stimulant have a important impact and can help these couples push through their low moments, maintain their stopgap, and continue working towards their dream of having a family. occasionally, the couple may need an outside source of stimulant, and that is where support groups, family, and musketeers come by.

Gravidity support groups can be an excellent source of stimulant for infertile couples.

These groups produce a safe space for couples to express themselves, partake their gests , and gain support from others who understand what they're going through.

Another way gravidity couples can stay encouraged is by connecting with others who have dealt with gravidity and successfully conceived.

Hearing stories of other couples' success can significantly impact gravidity couples by showing them that it's possible to conceive and that everyone's trip is different.
Social media platforms similar as Instagram and Facebook offer community groups where people can connect, support, and encourage each other throughout their trip. tone- care is critical for gravidity couples to stay encouraged as well.
Gravidity can take a risk on one's psyche, so taking the time to relax and concentrate on tone- care can help couples recharge and stay motivated.

Strategies similar as exercise, contemplation, journaling, or remedy can help gravidity couples reduce stress and anxiety, ameliorate their mood, ameliorate their physical health, and, eventually, help them feel encouraged and auspicious about their trip towards generality.
It's inversely important to fete and admit the challenges of the gravidity trip. bummers along the way are natural, and couples should learn not to let them define their trip. Rather, they should use these lapses as an occasion to reframe their perspective and work on their managing strategies.

Gravidity doesn't define who they're as a person, and couples should concentrate on getting support from their loved bones
and espousing a positive mindset.
In addition, it's important to keep in mind that gravidity is an issue that affects both mates. Both individualities in the relationship should take care of themselves and support each other through the trip.
Regular communication between mates is essential in icing both sense supported and heard.

Talking about gravidity can be delicate, but it's pivotal to talk about the issue and work through it as a platoon. In conclusion, gravidity can leave couples feeling hopeless, defeated, and alone.
It's a long, grueling trip that requires strength, tolerance, and stimulant to stay positive and motivated.

Gravidity couples can overcome this handicap by staying hopeful, talking to those who understand their situation, seeking tone- care, and feting that this trip is different for everyone.
Incipiently, above everything differently, they should have faith in themselves and each other because with stopgap, perseverance and lots of love, they can overcome gravidity.
As the notorious quotation goes," Where there's love, there's life" – so hold on tight to the love that brought you together.